CORE LIBRARY GUIDE TO COVID-19

UNDERSTANDING
COVID-19

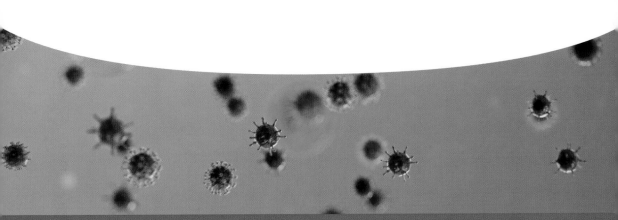

BY DOUGLAS HUSTAD

CONTENT CONSULTANT
Mark N. Lurie, PhD
Associate Professor of Epidemiology, International Health Institute
Brown University School of Public Health

Cover image: SARS-CoV-2 is a coronavirus that causes COVID-19.

Core Library

An Imprint of Abdo Publishing
abdobooks.com

abdobooks.com

Published by Abdo Publishing, a division of ABDO, PO Box 398166, Minneapolis, Minnesota 55439.
Copyright © 2021 by Abdo Consulting Group, Inc. International copyrights reserved in all countries.
No part of this book may be reproduced in any form without written permission from the publisher.
Core Library™ is a trademark and logo of Abdo Publishing.

Printed in the United States of America, North Mankato, Minnesota
072020
092020

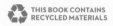

Cover Photo: iStockphoto
Interior Photos: iStockphoto, 4–5, 39; Shepherd Zhou/FeatureChina/AP Images, 6, 45; Alissa Eckert,
MS; Dan Higgins, MAMS/Public Health Image Library/CDC, 8; PA Images/Getty Images, 12–13; SDI
Productions/iStockphoto, 14; Shutterstock Images, 16, 18, 22, 24, 28, 32–33; May James /SOPA
Images/Sipa USA/AP Images, 20; SPL/Science Source, 27; Seth Wenig/AP Images, 34, 43; John
Minchillo/AP Images, 37

Editor: Angela Lim
Series Designer: Jake Nordby

Library of Congress Control Number: 2020936523

Publisher's Cataloging-in-Publication Data

Names: Hustad, Douglas, author.
Title: Understanding COVID-19 / by Douglas Hustad
Description: Minneapolis, Minnesota : Abdo Publishing, 2021 | Series: Core library guide to
    COVID-19 | Includes online resources and index
Identifiers: ISBN 9781532194078 (lib. bdg.) | ISBN 9781644945049 (pbk.) | ISBN 9781098212988
    (ebook)
Subjects: LCSH: Immunotechnology--Juvenile literature. | Medical technology--Juvenile literature.
    | Biomedical research--Juvenile literature. | Epidemics--Juvenile literature. | Communicable
    diseases--Prevention--Juvenile literature. | Health--Juvenile literature. | COVID-19 (Disease)--
    Juvenile literature.
Classification: DDC 614.54--dc23

CONTENTS

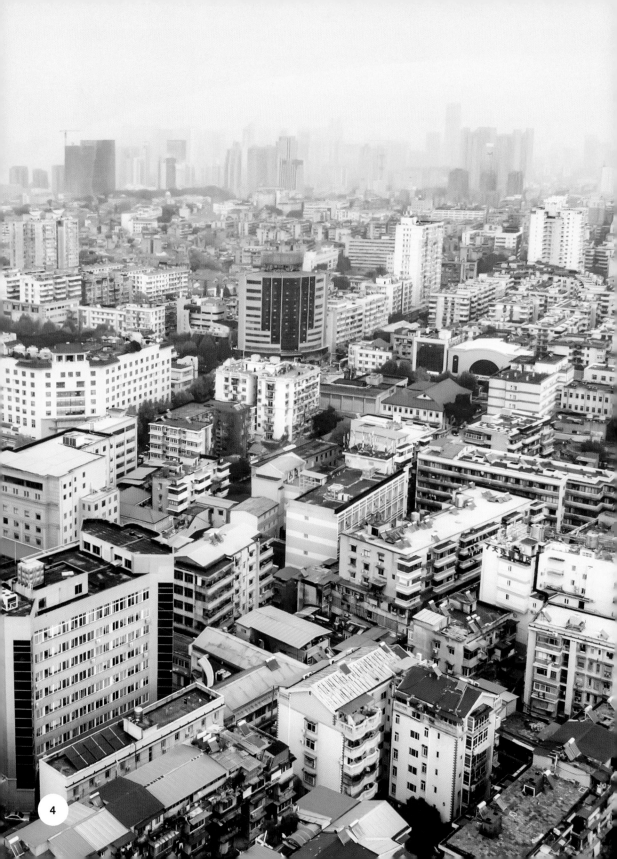

A MYSTERIOUS DISEASE

Wei Guixian began to feel sick on December 10, 2019. The 57-year-old shrimp vendor worked at a seafood market in Wuhan, China. At first the illness didn't seem serious. It felt like a regular cold. Wei took some medicine and went back to work.

In just over a week, she was in the hospital. She recovered in early January. But others in Wuhan were hospitalized with similar symptoms. They had fevers and coughs.

The earliest known cases of COVID-19 were in Wuhan, China. The disease was first linked to a local seafood market.

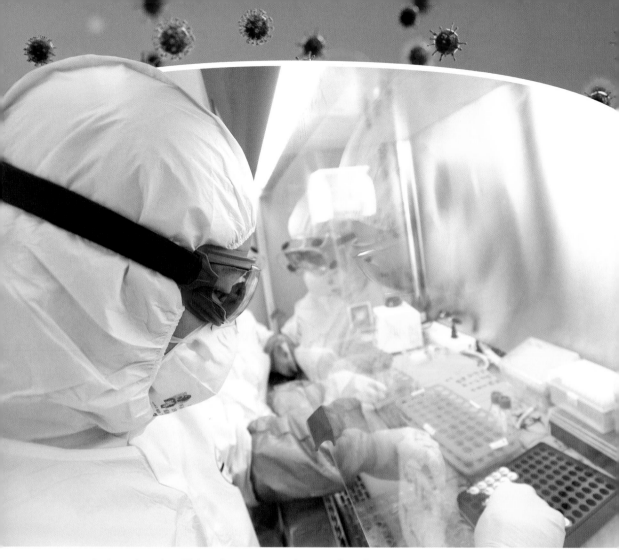

Scientists in China began studying the disease soon after the outbreak in Wuhan.

Some had difficulty breathing. Doctors didn't know what was causing the illness.

The Chinese government thought it was a new strain of pneumonia. The government believed it came from a Wuhan market. Scientists began to investigate the market. They wanted to understand this new disease.

Most of the first 41 patients had a connection to the market. Some worked there. Others shopped there. The market sold all kinds of meat. Some of the meat came from exotic animals that could carry disease. However, 13 of the patients had no connection to the market. The source of the disease was a mystery.

A GROWING THREAT

By late December, scientists realized this was not pneumonia. The disease resembled severe acute respiratory syndrome (SARS). SARS caused an outbreak in China in 2002. The disease spread to many countries and killed hundreds of people worldwide.

SARS belongs to a family of viruses called coronaviruses. These viruses have a telltale shape. They have long spiky rods that stick out from the surface. These rods can attach to human cells and cause

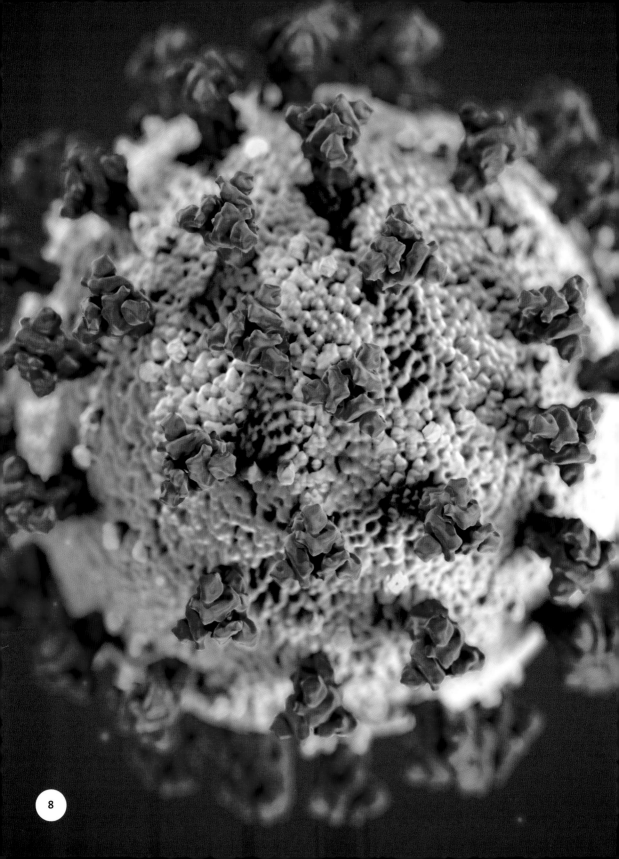

illnesses. The new virus also had this shape. Doctors would eventually name this virus SARS-CoV-2. The disease caused by the virus would soon be known as COVID-19.

Doctors in Wuhan reported their findings to the government. They warned that the new disease was like SARS. It could also spread quickly. The virus could kill a lot of people. But the Chinese government did not confirm it was dealing with a coronavirus until January 9.

CORONAVIRUSES

Coronaviruses get their names from Latin. *Corona* is the Latin word for "crown." When viewed under a microscope, the virus looks like a crown. The word *virus* is also Latin. It means "venom," which is a kind of poison. A virus is a tiny, disease-causing agent that can only survive inside a living host. *Coronavirus* refers to any member of a large family of viruses.

All coronaviruses have a similar shape. Each kind has many rods sticking out of its surface.

PERSPECTIVES

DR. LI WENLIANG

Dr. Li Wenliang was an eye doctor in Wuhan. He noticed how the disease affected his patients. Li tried to warn others about it on social media in late December. But the Chinese government censored his posts. This prevented important information about the virus from spreading. Soon afterward, Li got the disease from one of his patients. Li was in the hospital on January 20 when China first called the disease an emergency. The government apologized to him, but it was too late. Li died on February 7. He was hailed as a hero for speaking out about the disease.

That same day, the first known death from the new disease was recorded. The disease was still unnamed at the time. The World Health Organization (WHO) and the rest of the world were playing catch-up. Countries had to act fast to understand and contain this new global threat.

STRAIGHT TO THE
SOURCE

The WHO helped countries respond to the outbreak. An article on the WHO's website discussed what researchers do when they discover a new virus:

> *When a new virus is discovered, it is important to understand where it comes from. This is critical to be able to . . . prevent further introductions of the virus into the human population. It also helps to understand the dynamic of the beginning of the outbreak, which can be used to inform the public health response. Understanding the origin of the virus may also aid the development of therapeutics and vaccines.*
>
> *To identify the source or origin of a virus, it is helpful to look at the genetic makeup of the virus and see whether it resembles other known viruses. . . . Viruses that are genetically closely linked tend to come from a similar source or similar geographic area.*
>
> Source: "Origin of SARS-CoV-2: 26 March 2020." *World Health Organization*, 26 Mar. 2020, who.int. Accessed 8 Apr. 2020.

WHAT'S THE BIG IDEA?

Take a close look at this passage. Why is finding the source of the virus helpful in finding a cure? What evidence is used to support this?

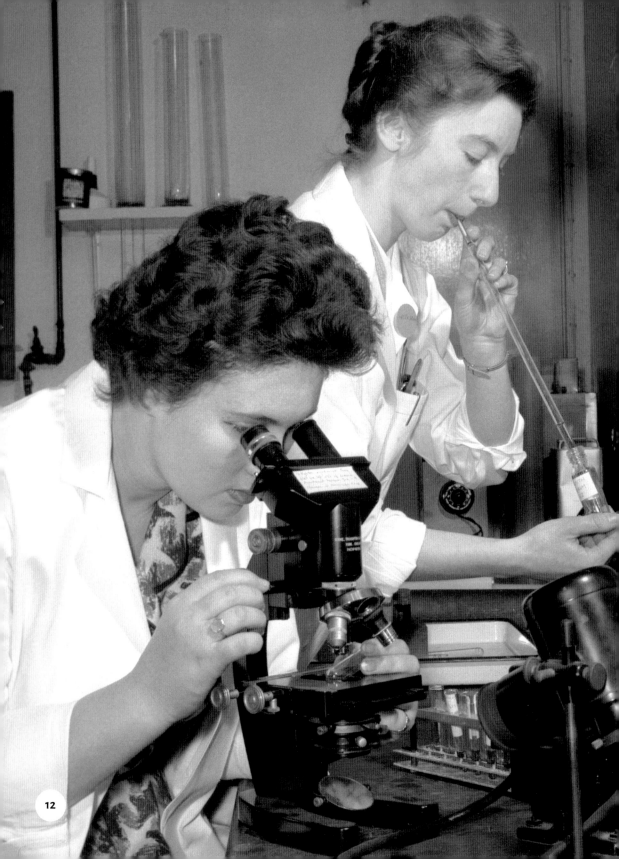

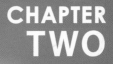

A NEW VIRUS

S cientists have been studying coronaviruses and the diseases they cause since the 1930s. These viruses were first seen in chickens. Human coronaviruses were discovered in the 1960s.

Only a few human coronaviruses were known before the 2002 SARS outbreak. Some of these viruses are widespread. Coronavirus 229E causes the common cold. Up to 30 percent of colds are caused by this virus. It infects millions of people each year.

Scientists at the Common Cold Research Unit in Salisbury, United Kingdom, discovered that the common cold can be caused by a coronavirus.

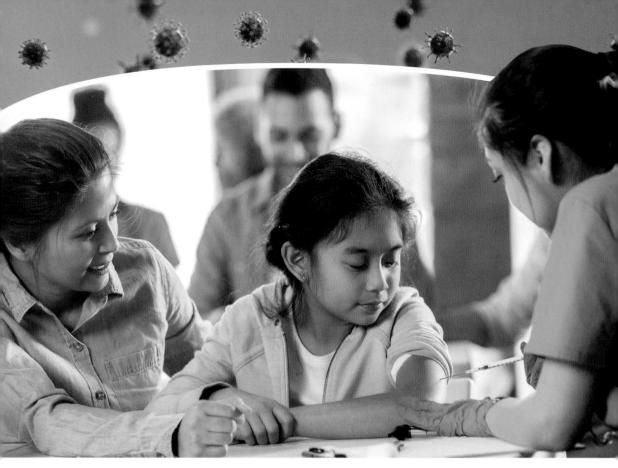

A vaccine introduces a person's immune system to a specific virus. It can protect a person from that virus in the future.

There are no cures for viruses. Vaccines can keep people from getting sick and prevent viral infections. Or the body's immune system can fight the virus off naturally. Some medicines and treatments help the immune system. They relieve symptoms and make people feel better.

Coronaviruses infect the lungs and other parts of the body that control breathing. They usually cause mild symptoms similar to a cold. But symptoms can also be very serious and cause breathing difficulties. A person may develop pneumonia. They may have to receive care in a hospital.

NAMING A VIRUS

COVID-19 went weeks without an official name. Some people called the disease the Wuhan virus or Chinese virus because that is where the virus was first discovered. But these names can cause people to react negatively to people of an East Asian background. The WHO avoids naming viruses after places. It changed its rules after MERS was already named. COVID-19 was named scientifically. *CO* stands for "corona." *VI* stands for "virus." The *D* is for "disease," and 19 is for the year it was discovered, 2019.

OTHER CORONAVIRUSES

A few recent outbreaks of coronaviruses have been deadly. The SARS outbreak of 2002 to 2004 killed hundreds of people. Middle East Respiratory Syndrome (MERS) has had several small outbreaks since it first

A CORONAVIRUS

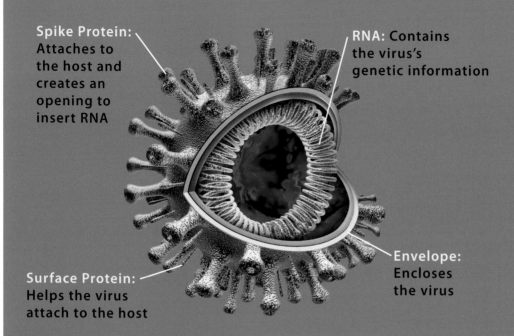

Spike Protein: Attaches to the host and creates an opening to insert RNA

RNA: Contains the virus's genetic information

Surface Protein: Helps the virus attach to the host

Envelope: Encloses the virus

A coronavirus is recognizable by its long, spiky rods. These rods let viruses attach to a host cell. Other parts of a coronavirus are also important. These features help coronaviruses infect people. The RNA carries genetic information. This information is used to make copies of the coronavirus within an infected cell. Then these copies can infect more cells. How does this image help you understand how coronaviruses infect people?

appeared in 2012. It also has killed hundreds. Both of these coronaviruses have high death rates. MERS kills more than 30 percent of the people it infects. The death rate for COVID-19 was still unknown as it began spreading around the world. Scientists estimated approximately 1 percent of cases are deadly.

But thousands more people have died from COVID-19 than from SARS and MERS combined. This is because SARS and MERS are less contagious. Fewer people were infected. COVID-19 is dangerous because of how easily it spreads. The SARS outbreak infected fewer than 10,000 people worldwide. COVID-19 infected millions within a few months.

The virus that causes SARS is known as SARS-CoV. COVID-19 is caused by SARS-CoV-2. The viruses are closely related. That is why the virus that causes COVID-19 was given a similar name.

SARS and MERS provide information to scientists. The virus that causes COVID-19 could infect others in a similar way. That helps scientists determine where it came from. They can then learn how to treat the illness.

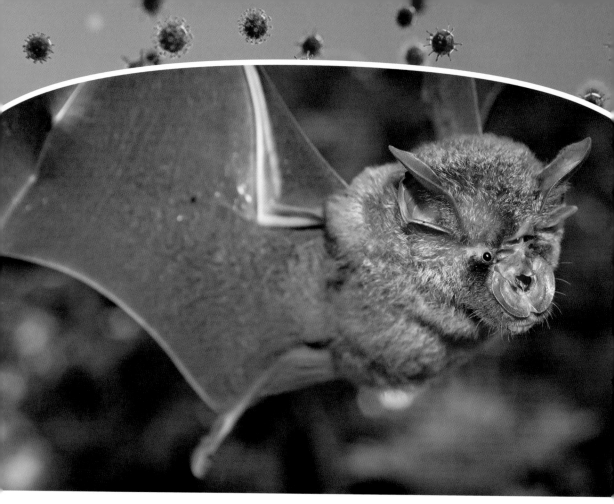

The coronavirus that caused SARS first came from bats. SARS-CoV-2 is also thought to be linked with bats.

AN ANIMAL HOST?

Human coronaviruses are closely linked to viruses in animals. The MERS virus can be traced to camels. The SARS virus originated in horseshoe bats. It was then passed to a catlike animal called a civet. Some people who touched sick civets became sick with SARS.

It is likely that COVID-19 also came from bats. But scientists aren't sure how the virus infected humans. The virus could have passed directly from bats to humans. It also could have passed through another animal. One theory was that the disease was carried by pangolins.

Pangolins are small animals that look like scaly anteaters. It is against international law to sell pangolins. But they are often sold illegally. Some people

PERSPECTIVES

DR. JONATHAN RUNSTADLER

COVID-19 can be tricky to diagnose. Its symptoms are similar to those of the flu. Dr. Jonathan Runstadler is a professor who researches the flu. He believes unfamiliarity with COVID-19 could be dangerous. People might not understand how serious it is. They may not take measures to protect themselves. This allows the disease to spread. "There were local outbreaks or minor epidemics of different flu strains in parts of Asia that didn't ultimately blow up into a pandemic," Runstadler said. "This is a different virus that we're much less familiar with—and that may be all the difference."

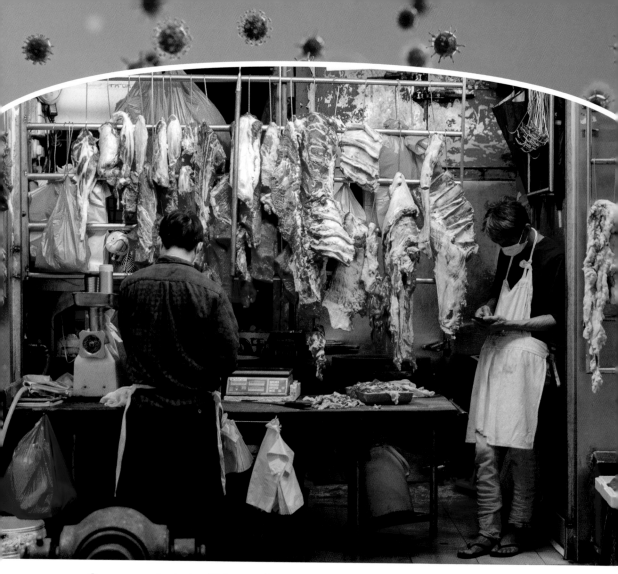

Some markets in China sell exotic meats and live animals. This type of environment can spread diseases.

believe pangolin scales can be used as medicine. The Wuhan seafood market sells live animals. If pangolins were illegally sold there, it could explain why the outbreak started there.

Markets like the Wuhan seafood market can be dangerous. These markets are not always kept clean. Different exotic animals are crowded together. Diseases may spread between the animals. A disease might even infect a person.

Scientists believed these conditions allowed SARS-CoV-2 to spread to humans. At first, the Chinese government did not realize how dangerous the virus was. Its response to the outbreak came too late. The virus had already begun to spread around the world.

FURTHER EVIDENCE

Chapter Two discusses how the virus that causes COVID-19 is similar to and different from other viruses. Review the information in this chapter. Then go to the website below. Find a quote that supports this chapter's main point. Does the website offer any other supporting information? Does it offer any new evidence?

HOW THE VIRUS THAT CAUSES COVID-19 DIFFERS FROM OTHER CORONAVIRUSES

abdocorelibrary.com/understanding-covid-19

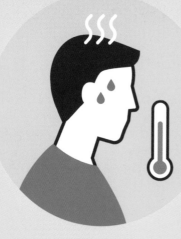

FEVER

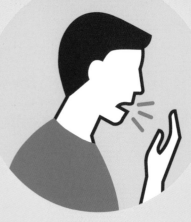

COUGH

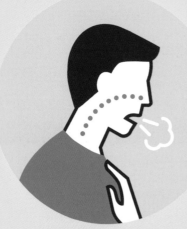

SHORTNESS OF BREATH

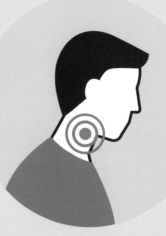

SORE THROAT

HEADACHE

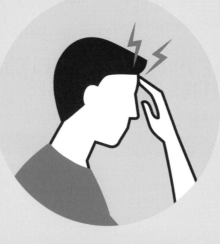

SYMPTOMS AND TRANSMISSION

Symptoms of COVID-19 vary from person to person. The most common symptoms include fever, coughing, and shortness of breath. People may also feel tired or have body aches. They may have a sore throat. Rarer symptoms include loss of smell or taste.

These symptoms may take days or weeks to appear. Most people show symptoms within two to 14 days after contact with a person who has COVID-19. This contact is known as exposure. Symptoms are usually mild.

Common symptoms of COVID-19 include coughing and a fever.

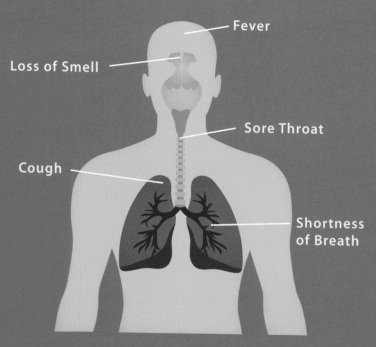

COVID-19 SYMPTOMS

Fever

Loss of Smell

Sore Throat

Cough

Shortness of Breath

COVID-19 is a respiratory illness. This means that areas of the body that help with breathing are affected. COVID-19 patients usually describe symptoms in their throat and lungs. Sometimes these symptoms can become very serious. People might have trouble breathing. They have to be treated in hospitals. How does this image help you understand how COVID-19 affects the respiratory system?

Some people do not show symptoms at all. But they can still spread the virus.

Anybody can become sick from the virus. Nobody is more likely to get it than anybody else. But the virus is more dangerous to certain groups of people. The virus attacks the lungs. The disease is more severe for people with breathing problems. People with weak immune systems also have more problems fighting the virus. This includes older people. Older people usually have more severe symptoms. The symptoms in young people tend to be mild. Young people are also less likely to die from the disease.

The United States had the most COVID-19 cases in the world by April 2020. At that time, 78 percent of American deaths were

PERSPECTIVES

JONAH STILLMAN

The COVID-19 virus can be dangerous for older people. But it can infect anyone. Even younger people can become seriously ill. That was the case for 20-year-old Jonah Stillman of Excelsior, Minnesota. At first, Stillman had mild symptoms. "I had a tiny cough and sore throat," he said. But after a few days, he quickly felt worse. "I went from having what felt like a head cold to high fever, the worst body aches I've ever had," he said. "It felt like I was in a horrible car accident almost. I couldn't move. . . . The simplest of tasks would wind me."

of people 65 or over. But every age group had at least one reported death.

ONSET OF INFECTION

COVID-19 has a dangerous effect on the lungs. The virus enters the body through the nose, mouth, and eyes. It attaches to cells and multiplies. The virus makes copies of itself. These copies infect more healthy cells.

The virus travels into the lungs. The immune system tries to fight the virus. This causes the lungs and airways to swell.

In serious cases, the virus infects both lungs. Fluid is created as the body fights the disease. The lungs might fill with this fluid and cause pneumonia. This makes it difficult to breathe. The lungs are unable to take in enough oxygen. This can be especially deadly for patients who already have lung problems such as asthma.

The immune response to COVID-19 can lead to fluid buildup in the lungs. This buildup, which is seen as a yellow blob in this X-ray, causes pneumonia.

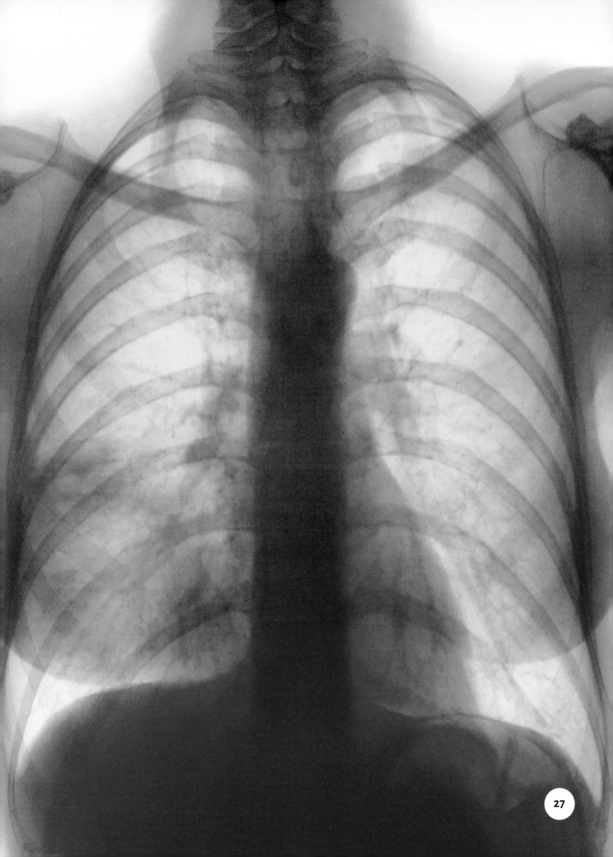

COVID-19 PREVENTION

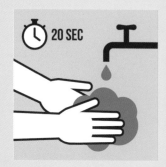

WASH HANDS WITH WATER AND SOAP/SANITIZER, AT LEAST 20 SECONDS

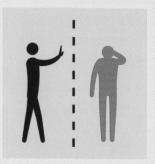

AVOID CONTACT WITH SICK PEOPLE

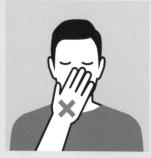

DON'T TOUCH EYES, NOSE, OR MOUTH WITH UNWASHED HANDS

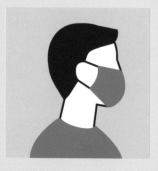

WEAR A MASK

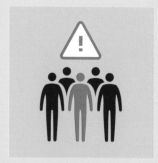

AVOID CROWDED PLACES

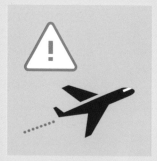

AVOID TRAVELING TO AFFECTED AREAS UNLESS NECESSARY

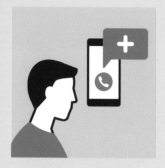

IF YOU BECOME SERIOUSLY ILL, SEEK MEDICAL CARE

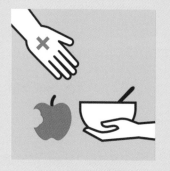

DO NOT SHARE EATING UTENSILS AND FOOD

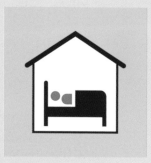

STAY AT HOME

In healthy people, the disease is usually mild. Most people recover. Some may have a lingering cough. Other long-term effects will only be known with time.

TRANSMISSION

The virus that causes COVID-19 is most often spread through the air. Infected people cough. The virus leaves the body in droplets. These droplets can land on nearby people. The virus directly enters the body if it lands on an opening such as the mouth. Or it could land on a person's hand. That person could then touch his or her mouth or eyes and become infected.

The virus does not live in the air for long. The droplets are too heavy to stay airborne. That means the virus does not remain in the air people breathe.

The droplets could fall onto a surface. The amount of time the virus can stay on a surface varies. But it can stay on some surfaces for a few days. People could touch this surface and then rub their eyes. They could

There are many ways to prevent getting sick with COVID-19.

get infected. This is a rare form of infection. Most cases are spread directly from person to person.

MISINFORMATION

Information changes quickly during a pandemic. People might not always be getting the right message. This led to conspiracy theories about where the virus came from. Some people suggested the virus was created to be used as a weapon. But scientists studied the virus closely. A human-made virus must be based on other known viruses. But there were characteristics of SARS-CoV-2 that had never been seen before. It would have been impossible to generate this virus in a lab.

Symptoms can appear two to 14 days after exposure. But it is possible to spread the disease before symptoms appear. Some research indicated people may be highly infectious during the days before they develop symptoms. For this reason, people who did not feel sick were still told to follow safety procedures.

Scientists continue to study the symptoms and spread of COVID-19. They want to learn as much as they can about the virus. New information can help patients.

EXPLORE ONLINE

Chapter Three discusses some of the common symptoms of COVID-19. This website from the Centers for Disease Control and Prevention helps people check themselves for symptoms of the disease. Review the information on the site. Compare and contrast that with the information in this chapter. How is it the same? How is it different?

SYMPTOMS OF CORONAVIRUS

abdocorelibrary.com/understanding-covid-19

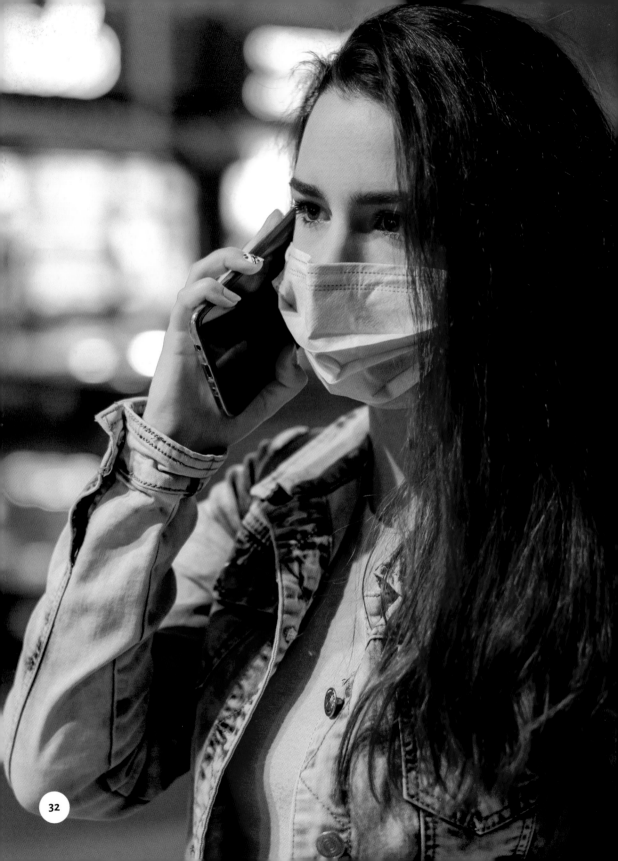

TESTING AND TREATMENT

Being aware of COVID-19 symptoms is important. People can wear masks and take other steps to prevent spreading the disease if they feel sick. But COVID-19 shares symptoms with many other diseases. A medical test is the only way to diagnose COVID-19.

A new test was needed to detect the virus. Testing was not widely available at first. This was a problem for several reasons. People did not know if they had the disease. This meant

Wearing a mask prevents droplets from spreading to others. It can also protect the wearer from getting infected.

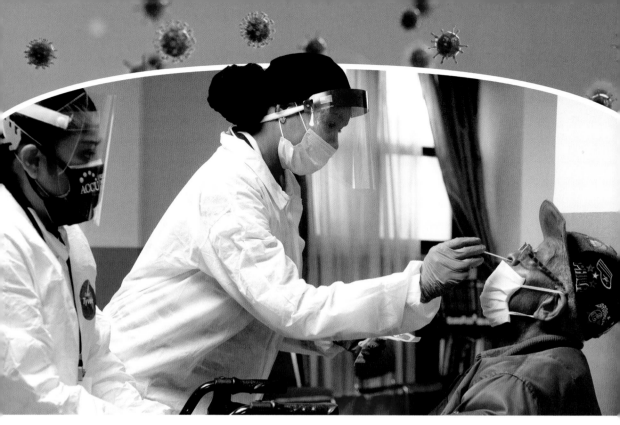

Doctors tested residents in senior housing to make sure they were not infected with SARS-CoV-2.

that many did not isolate themselves. They could infect others. Without widespread testing, it was difficult to determine if progress was being made in containing the disease.

There are two kinds of COVID-19 tests. One test looks for active infection. This means the person has the disease at the time of the test. A swab is used to take a sample from the back of the nose and throat. The swab is studied in a lab. Results are available in a couple of days.

Another test is a serological test. This test looks for antibodies. Antibodies might not be present in the early stages of COVID-19. So serological tests aren't used for diagnosis. They show who has had the disease. This helps track the spread.

Scientists do not know whether people who recover from COVID-19 become immune to the disease. But they believe immunity is a possibility. If a serological test can show who has had the disease, those people may no longer have

REINFECTION

Scientists wanted to know if those who recovered from COVID-19 would be immune to the disease. With some viruses, having the disease once makes people immune to it in the future. Someone who recovers from measles cannot get measles a second time. Patients with MERS were less likely to get the disease again. But immunity to COVID-19 was still unknown. Scientists studied antibodies to determine whether people can get reinfected with SARS-CoV-2.

to fear exposure. That knowledge plays a key role in responding to the disease.

TREATMENT

There is no cure for a virus. COVID-19 is treated by reducing the symptoms. Most cases of COVID-19 are mild. People do not have to go to the hospital. They should stay home, rest, and drink plenty of water. Basic medicines such as Tylenol (acetaminophen) can help with fever and aches.

Scientists studied new drugs to help treat COVID-19. The antiviral drug remdesivir was approved for emergency use in the United States on May 1, 2020. Scientists in the United Kingdom researched the drug dexamethasone. This drug helped one-third of patients with severe cases of COVID-19 to recover.

Severe cases of COVID-19 require more care. People who are having trouble breathing are taken to a hospital's intensive care unit (ICU). They receive oxygen from a mask.

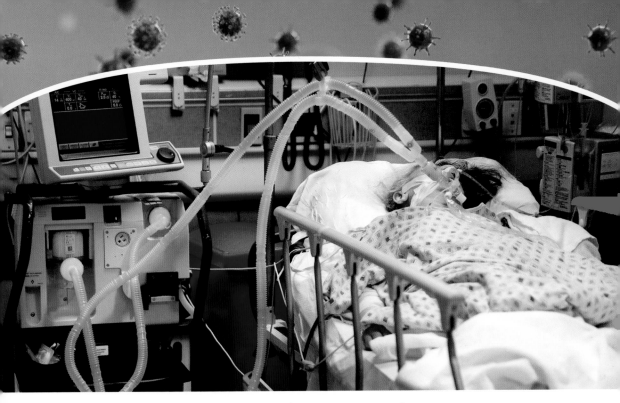

Patients with severe cases of COVID-19 may be put on a ventilator. This machine helps patients breathe.

If that doesn't help, a patient is intubated. This procedure places a tube into the throat. The tube is hooked up to a machine called a ventilator, which breathes for the patient. Patients at this stage are seriously ill. Sometimes a ventilator is not enough to fight off the disease.

In addition to tests, ventilators were necessary items in short supply during the pandemic. Hospitals do not normally need many. But they suddenly needed thousands of them. Overcoming this problem was essential to saving lives.

PREVENTION

As hospitals filled with patients, scientists were still working on a vaccine to prevent the disease. Early detection of the disease was the best way to prevent further spread. People who tested positive for COVID-19 were isolated so they could not infect others.

There are other steps that reduce the risk of getting sick. World leaders recommended keeping 6 feet (1.8 m) between people. This lowers the risk of droplets spreading from person to person.

Hand washing is a simple way to stay safe. Soap splits the protective layer around the virus. Then the virus can no longer infect people. Twenty seconds of hand washing can destroy the virus. People also cleaned surfaces whenever possible.

Scientists hoped to develop a vaccine that would prevent people from becoming infected. A vaccine

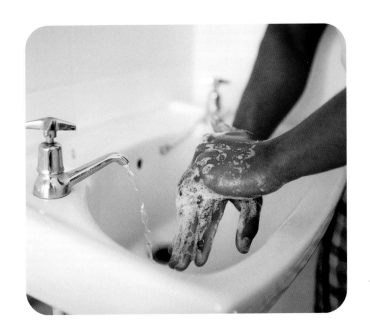

Health officials reminded people to wash their hands with soap for at least 20 seconds. This destroys the virus and prevents the spread of disease.

is a medicine made from a weakened form of a virus. It is injected into the body. The vaccine is not strong enough to make someone sick. The body responds to the vaccine by making antibodies. These antibodies help the body recognize the same virus in the future. It is then prepared to fight it off.

Vaccines are not easy to create. They take a long time to develop. And they need to be tested many times to prove that they are safe and effective. COVID-19 vaccine research only began in early 2020. Scientists estimated it would take at least a year to

18 months to make a vaccine for COVID-19. Vaccines usually take even longer to develop.

PERSPECTIVES

HANNEKE SCHUITEMAKER

Making a vaccine can be a long and difficult process. Hanneke Schuitemaker is the head vaccine scientist for a company that makes vaccines. A vaccine has to go through trials. Scientists need to make sure it is safe. "For it to work we will have to give it to healthy people in the knowledge that they may never actually encounter the virus," she said. "In other words, they may never benefit from the vaccine's protection yet they could be put at risk from potential side effects. So you will have to be very sure that your vaccine is safe in such circumstances."

Fighting COVID-19 was like aiming at a moving target. Information changed quickly. And the virus continued to spread to more people. That is why it was important to learn more about the virus. Scientists could use information about where the virus came from, whom it infects, and how it spreads to prevent further infections of COVID-19.

STRAIGHT TO THE
SOURCE

Dr. Eduardo Sanchez is the chief medical officer for prevention with the American Heart Association. In this passage, he expands on the importance of testing:

When a communicable disease outbreak begins, the ideal response is for public health officials to begin testing for it early. That leads to quick identification of cases, quick treatment for those people and immediate isolation to prevent spread. Early testing also helps to identify anyone who came into contact with infected people so they too can be quickly treated. . . .

It's crucial of course to help treat . . . people who are infected. Testing . . . help[s] investigators characterize the prevalence, spread and contagiousness of the disease.

Source: Eduardo Sanchez. "COVID-19 Science: Why Testing Is So Important." *American Heart Association*, 2 Apr. 2020, healthmetrics.heart.org. Accessed 17 Apr. 2020

CONSIDER YOUR AUDIENCE

Adapt this passage for a different audience, such as your group of friends. Write a blog post conveying this same information for the new audience. How does your post differ from the source text and why?

FAST FACTS

- COVID-19 is a disease caused by the virus SARS-CoV-2, a type of coronavirus that affects the human respiratory system.

- SARS-CoV-2 came from an animal before passing to humans, but its exact origin was hard for scientists to determine.

- The first known case of COVID-19 was identified in China in December 2019. The disease then began spreading around the world, causing millions of cases and thousands of deaths in 2020.

- Symptoms of COVID-19 commonly include fever, cough, and shortness of breath. It is spread through the air in droplets that infected people cough or sneeze outward. Many people experience only mild symptoms.

- There is no cure for COVID-19, but symptoms can be treated. In serious cases for patients having difficulty breathing, they may need oxygen or a ventilator.

- Long-term solutions to COVID-19 include developing a vaccine, but it is a process that can take a year or longer.

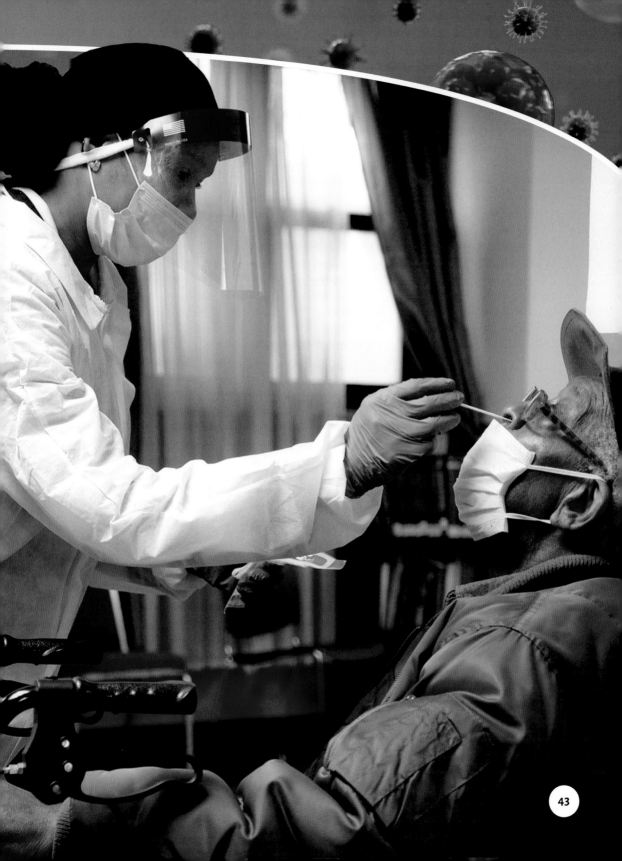

STOP AND
THINK

Why Do I Care?

Maybe you don't know anyone who has COVID-19. But that doesn't mean you shouldn't be educated about it. How does the health of others affect your life? In what ways does a pandemic affect everyone?

Dig Deeper

Chapter Two discusses the family of coronaviruses. After reading this book, what questions do you still have about these viruses? With an adult's help, find a few reliable sources that can help you answer your questions. Write a paragraph about what you learned.

Surprise Me

Chapter Three discusses the symptoms and transmission of COVID-19. After reading this book, what two or three facts about COVID-19 did you find the most surprising? Write a few sentences about each one. Why did you find these facts surprising?

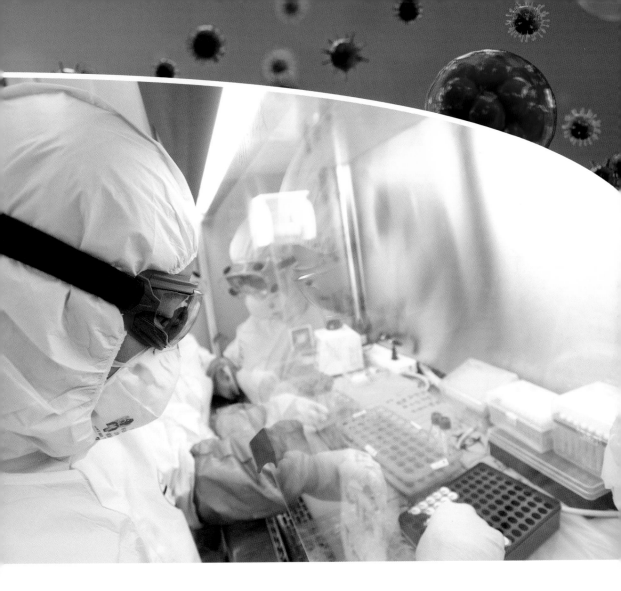

You Are There

Imagine you have a friend who has a fever and is coughing. Using the information you learned in this book, what advice would you give your friend so that they don't get others sick?

GLOSSARY

censor
to block or prevent information from being seen

communicable
able to be spread

conspiracy theory
an idea that the truth about something is different from the official explanation

contagious
able to be spread to other people

immune system
the body's natural defense against disease

immunity
being protected from getting a certain disease

microscope
a device for magnifying tiny things

outbreak
the sudden increase in cases of a disease

pneumonia
a serious respiratory disease

respiratory
having to do with the lungs and airways

side effect
a symptom a person experiences as a result of taking a medication

ONLINE RESOURCES

To learn more about COVID-19, visit our free resource websites below.

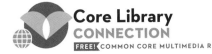

Visit **abdocorelibrary.com** or scan this QR code for free Common Core resources for teachers and students, including vetted activities, multimedia, and booklinks, for deeper subject comprehension.

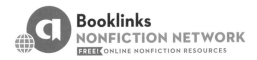

Visit **abdobooklinks.com** or scan this QR code for free additional online weblinks for further learning. These links are routinely monitored and updated to provide the most current information available.

LEARN MORE

Alkire, Jessie. *Medicine: From Hippocrates to Jonas Salk*. Abdo Publishing, 2019.

London, Martha. *The Spread of COVID-19*. Abdo Publishing, 2021.

INDEX

About the Author

Douglas Hustad is a freelance writer and author of dozens of science and history books for young people. He and his family live in northern San Diego County.